COMPLETE GUIDE TO GASTRITIS

Definitive Handbook For Understanding, Prevention, Healing Strategies For Digestive Wellness, Essential Remedies, Diet Plans, And Natural Relief Methods Included

DEHART HAIRSTON

© [DEHART HAIRSTON], [2024]

All rights reserved. No part of this publication may be reproduced, distributed, or transmitted in any form or by any means, including photocopying, recording, or other electronic or mechanical methods, without the prior written permission of the publisher, except in the case of brief quotations embodied in critical reviews and certain other noncommercial uses permitted by copyright law.

DISCLAIMER

This book's content is only intended for general informative purposes. At the time of writing, the author has taken every precaution to guarantee that the material is correct and current. Nevertheless, the author disclaims all explicit and implicit representations and guarantees about the availability, appropriateness, correctness, completeness, and usefulness of the material on these pages.

Since the author is not a licensed medical practitioner, the material in this book shouldn't be interpreted as medical advice. Before making any modifications to their diet, exercise regimen, or medical treatment, readers are urged to speak with a licensed healthcare provider.

Moreover, the author has no connection to any of the businesses, organizations, or people that are discussed in this book. Any mentions of goods, services, businesses, or people are purely informative and do not indicate endorsement or suggestion.

This book's content is entirely dependent on the author's expertise, study, and comprehension of the topic. Despite having taken reasonable care to offer correct information, the author disclaims all liability for any mistakes or omissions in the material as well as for any losses, harm, or damages resulting from using the information.

It is recommended that readers use their own judgment and discretion when applying the knowledge in this book to their own situations. The use or implementation of any material in this book may result in unfavorable repercussions, directly or indirectly, for which the author assumes no liability.

By reading this book, you agree to release and hold the author harmless from any claims, losses, liabilities, costs, or expenditures resulting from or related to the use of the information you get from it.

Table of Contents

CHAPTER 1 13
Understanding Gastritis 13
What Is Gastritis? 13
Causes Of Gastritis 14
- 1. Helicobacter pylori Infection: 14
- 5. Stress: 15
- 6. Autoimmune Diseases: 15

Symptoms Of Gastritis 16
- 1. Abdominal discomfort or Discomfort: 16
- 2. Nausea and Vomiting: 17
- 3. Indigestion: 17
- 4. Loss of Appetite: 17
- 5. Hematemesis or Melena: 17
- 6. Heartburn: 17

CHAPTER 2 19
Types Of Gastritis 19
Acute Gastritis 19
Chronic Gastritis 20
Erosive Gastritis 21
Atrophic Gastritis 22

CHAPTER 3 25
  Diagnosis Of Gastritis 25
  Medical History And Physical Examination 25
  Endoscopy 26
  Biopsy 26
  Blood Tests 27
CHAPTER 4 29
  Lifestyle Changes For Managing Gastritis 29
  Dietary Guidelines 29
  Stress Management Techniques 31
  Avoiding Irritants 33
  Importance Of Adequate Sleep 35
CHAPTER 5 37
  Medications For Gastritis 37
  Antacids 37
  Proton Pump Inhibitors (Ppis) 38
  H2 Receptor Blockers 39
  Antibiotics (For H. Pylori Infection) 40
CHAPTER 6 43
  Herbal Remedies And Natural Treatments 43
  Aloe Vera 43

Ginger 44

Licorice Root 45

Probiotics 46

CHAPTER 7 48

Preventing Gastritis Flare-Ups 48

Maintaining A Healthy Diet 48

Stress Reduction Strategies 50

Limiting Alcohol And Caffeine Intake 52

Avoiding Smoking 53

CHAPTER 8 56

Complications Of Gastritis 56

Peptic Ulcers 56

Gastric Cancer 58

Anemia 59

Malabsorption 61

CHAPTER 9 64

Gastritis In Special Populations 64

Gastritis In Children 64

Causes 64

Symptoms 65

Diagnosis 65

Treatment 66

Prevention 66

Gastritis During Pregnancy 67

Causes 67

Symptoms 67

Diagnosis 68

Treatment 68

Gastritis In The Elderly 69

Causes 69

Symptoms 70

Diagnosis 70

Treatment 71

Prevention 71

CHAPTER 10 74

Living Well With Gastritis 74

Long-Term Management Strategies 74

Coping With Flare-Ups 75

Support Networks And Resources 77

Importance Of Regular Check-Ups 78

CONCLUSION 80

THE END 83

ABOUT THIS BOOK

"Gastritis" is more than simply a medical book; it is a thorough guide that can change the lives of those suffering from gastrointestinal pain. In today's environment, when lifestyle-related diseases are on the increase, understanding and properly controlling gastritis is critical to overall health.

Chapter 1 lays the groundwork by defining gastritis, its causes, and the warning indications to look out for. Understanding the complexities of this ailment enables people to proactively manage their health. Chapter 2 discusses the numerous kinds of gastritis, including acute, chronic, erosive, and atrophic gastritis, each of which necessitates a unique therapy strategy.

Diagnosis is critical, and Chapter 3 describes the methods required, from medical history to sophisticated tests such as endoscopy and biopsy.

Individuals with this understanding may seek immediate assistance. The lifestyle changes outlined in Chapter 4 serve as cornerstones for controlling gastritis, stressing dietary changes, stress management measures, and the necessity of getting enough sleep.

In Chapter 5, this book guides readers through the labyrinth of drugs, including information on antacids, proton pump inhibitors, H2 receptor blockers, and antibiotics, giving them a full arsenal for relief. But the trip does not end there. Chapter 6 covers herbal cures and natural therapies, providing options for people who choose holistic care.

Prevention is usually better than treatment, and Chapter 7 discusses tactics for avoiding gastritis flare-ups while also fostering gut health behaviors. Chapter 8 discusses possible consequences and emphasizes the importance of untreated gastritis. Chapters 9 and 10 focus on specific populations and long-term management, promoting inclusion and sustainability in health practices.

This book is more than simply facts; it is also about empowerment. With the information included inside its pages, readers may confidently navigate their gastritis journey, making educated choices, reducing risks, and adopting a digestively healthy lifestyle. Whether you're a sufferer, a caregiver, or a healthcare professional, "Gastritis" is an essential resource for achieving maximum gastrointestinal health.

CHAPTER 1

Understanding Gastritis

What Is Gastritis?

Gastritis is a frequent illness that causes inflammation of the stomach lining. This inflammation may develop immediately (acute gastritis) or gradually over time (chronic gastritis). The stomach lining includes unique cells that create acid and enzymes to facilitate digestion. When this lining gets irritated, it may cause a range of symptoms and pain.

Acute gastritis is often induced by irritants such as alcohol, certain medicines such as nonsteroidal anti-inflammatory drugs (NSAIDs), bacterial infections such as Helicobacter pylori, or stress. Chronic gastritis, on the other hand, might develop gradually as a result of frequent stomach lining irritation, autoimmune illnesses, or infections.

Causes Of Gastritis

Understanding the underlying causes of gastritis is critical for both therapy and prevention. Several factors may lead to the development of gastritis, including:

1. **Helicobacter pylori Infection:** This bacteria is one of the leading causes of gastritis. It may infect the stomach lining and cause inflammation, which, if not treated, can lead to ulcers or stomach cancer.

2. Nonsteroidal anti-inflammatory medicines (NSAIDs) such as aspirin, ibuprofen, and naproxen may irritate the stomach lining when used often or in large dosages. Long-term usage of these drugs is a leading cause of gastritis.

3. Excessive alcohol intake may irritate the stomach lining, resulting in inflammation. Chronic alcohol usage increases the likelihood of developing gastritis and other gastrointestinal issues.

4. Smoking may raise stomach acid levels and weaken the stomach's protective lining, leaving it more prone to irritation and injury.

5. **Stress:** While stress can not directly cause gastritis, it can aggravate pre-existing symptoms or contribute to the condition's development. Chronic stress may impair the immune system, increasing susceptibility to infections such as H. pylori.

6. **Autoimmune Diseases:** In certain situations, the immune system may erroneously target stomach lining cells, causing persistent inflammation and gastritis. Autoimmune gastritis is often connected with other autoimmune diseases, such as thyroid problems or type 1 diabetes.

7. Bile reflux occurs when bile, a digestive fluid generated by the liver, rushes backward into the stomach, irritating the stomach lining and causing inflammation. Bile reflux gastritis is more likely in

those who have had their gallbladder surgically removed.

Identifying the underlying cause of gastritis is critical for devising an effective treatment strategy and avoiding recurrences. In many situations, addressing lifestyle issues like food, medication usage, and stress management may aid in symptom reduction and recovery.

Symptoms Of Gastritis

Gastritis may cause a wide range of symptoms, from minor discomfort to extreme agony. Common symptoms of gastritis might include:

1. Abdominal discomfort or Discomfort: **Many people with gastritis have dull, gnawing discomfort or a burning feeling in their upper belly, especially after eating or drinking.**

2. **Nausea and Vomiting:** Gastritis may produce nausea, which may be followed by vomiting, particularly after ingesting irritating foods or drinks.

3. **Indigestion:** Some patients with gastritis may have indigestion or bloating, which is often accompanied by a sense of fullness or pain in the upper abdomen.

4. **Loss of Appetite:** Gastritis may reduce appetite and cause unexpected weight loss, especially if eating worsens symptoms.

5. **Hematemesis or Melena:** In severe instances of gastritis, inflammation of the stomach lining may cause bleeding. This may cause you to vomit blood (hematemesis) or produce black, tarry stools.

6. **Heartburn:** Many people with gastritis develop heartburn, which is a burning feeling in the chest or

neck produced by stomach acid refluxing into the esophagus.

7. Fatigue and weakness are common symptoms of chronic gastritis, which may be caused by food malabsorption or anemia caused by gastrointestinal hemorrhage.

Recognizing these signs is critical for early detection and treatment of gastritis. If you have chronic stomach discomfort, nausea, vomiting, or other concerns, you should see a doctor for an examination and treatment. Early management may assist people with gastritis to avoid problems and enhance their quality of life.

CHAPTER 2

Types Of Gastritis

Acute Gastritis

Acute gastritis is like a violent storm in the stomach, causing inflammation and irritation of the sensitive lining. It is often caused by a range of reasons, including spicy meals, heavy alcohol consumption, certain drugs like aspirin or ibuprofen, bacterial infections like H. Pylori, or even stress. Consider this scenario: you've had a feast of fiery tacos and washed it down with a few too many margaritas, and your stomach is rumbling!

Acute gastritis symptoms might include a burning feeling in the upper abdomen, nausea, vomiting, bloating, and even a lack of appetite. But don't worry, acute gastritis is generally short-lived and may be treated with easy measures such as avoiding irritants, eating bland meals, keeping hydrated, and using antacids for comfort. Consider it as enduring a storm; it may be difficult at first, but the sun will ultimately shine over your stomach landscape.

Chronic Gastritis

Chronic gastritis is more like a steady rain that wears away the stomach lining over time. Chronic gastritis, unlike acute gastritis, tends to last longer, frequently owing to continuous causes such as persistent infection with H. pylori bacteria, long-term use of certain drugs, immunological problems, or even the stomach's sensitivity to bile reflux. Consider the gradual loss of the stomach's protecting layers, making it exposed to pain and inflammation.

Chronic gastritis symptoms are less spectacular than those of acute gastritis, but they may be just as bothersome, with persistent stomach discomfort, bloating, nausea, and a sense of fullness after eating even modest quantities. controlling chronic gastritis requires a more long-term strategy that often includes lifestyle modifications such as avoiding irritants, eating a stomach-friendly diet, controlling stress, and, in some instances, drugs to lower stomach acid or cure underlying illnesses.

Erosive Gastritis

Erosive gastritis is similar to a storm surge, causing extensive destruction to the stomach lining. It is distinguished by the erosion of the stomach's mucous membrane, which leaves raw, exposed regions susceptible to additional injury and inflammation. This kind of gastritis may be induced by long-term use of nonsteroidal anti-inflammatory medicines (NSAIDs) such as aspirin or ibuprofen, excessive alcohol use, extreme stress, or even bile reflux.

Erosive gastritis symptoms may be severe, including strong stomach pain, recurrent vomiting (often with blood), black, tarry stools, and even indicators of bleeding like dizziness or fainting. Dealing with erosive gastritis needs immediate medical intervention to address the underlying cause and avoid more harm. Treatment may include quitting NSAIDs or alcohol, taking drugs to preserve the stomach lining, and, in extreme situations, doing an endoscopy to examine and treat the damage immediately.

Atrophic Gastritis

Atrophic gastritis is like a fading sunset; it progressively reduces the stomach's ability to operate normally. It is distinguished by the progressive loss of the stomach lining and the gastric glands, which generate vital digesting fluids such as hydrochloric acid and intrinsic factors. This kind of gastritis is often associated with chronic H.

infection. pylori bacteria, autoimmune diseases such as pernicious anemia, or even long-term inflammation from other sources.

Atrophic gastritis symptoms may not be visible right away since it usually develops gradually over time. However, when the stomach's capacity to generate digestive juices declines, it may cause symptoms such as indigestion, bloating, malabsorption of nutrients (leading to deficiencies such as vitamin B12), and an increased risk of developing stomach ulcers or even stomach cancer. Managing atrophic gastritis entails treating the underlying cause, such as H. pylori infection or vitamin B12 supplementation, as well as lifestyle adjustments that promote gut health. Regular monitoring and follow-up are critical for detecting problems early and ensuring appropriate treatment.

CHAPTER 3

Diagnosis Of Gastritis

Medical History And Physical Examination

A detailed medical history and physical examination are usually required to diagnose gastritis. Your doctor will inquire about your symptoms, particularly any pain or discomfort in your upper abdomen, nausea, vomiting, or changes in appetite. They will also ask about your medical history, including any past gastrointestinal problems or treatments.

During the physical examination, your doctor may gently touch your belly to detect pain or edema. They may also listen to your belly using a stethoscope for any unusual noises that might signal underlying digestive issues.

Endoscopy

Endoscopy is an important diagnostic technique for gastritis. During an endoscopy, a thin, flexible tube with a camera attached (endoscope) is passed via the mouth and into the esophagus, stomach, and duodenum. This enables the doctor to visually check the stomach lining for symptoms of inflammation, irritation, or ulcers.

Endoscopy is usually conducted with anesthesia to ensure the patient's comfort. It gives the doctor a clear view of the stomach lining, enabling him to examine the degree of gastritis and discover any other possible problems, such as bleeding or tumors.

Biopsy

During the endoscopy, the doctor may collect tiny samples of tissue from the stomach lining for biopsy.

These samples are transported to a laboratory to be examined under a microscope. A biopsy may assist confirm the diagnosis of gastritis and pinpoint the underlying cause, such as an H infection. pylori bacteria, or an autoimmune condition.

A biopsy may also help rule out more severe illnesses, such as stomach cancer. The treatment is rapid and safe, with a low chance of complications.

Blood Tests

Blood testing may help with the diagnosis of gastritis. Your doctor may prescribe blood tests to look for symptoms of infection, inflammation, or anemia. Blood testing may also show antibodies to the H. pylori bacterium is a frequent cause of gastritis.

In addition to these particular tests, your doctor may prescribe other blood tests to evaluate your general health and rule out any other possible reasons for your symptoms.

Your doctor may effectively diagnose gastritis by integrating information from your medical history, physical examination, endoscopy, biopsy, and blood tests and developing an appropriate treatment plan to alleviate your symptoms and address the underlying cause.

CHAPTER 4

Lifestyle Changes For Managing Gastritis

Dietary Guidelines

Diet is an important factor in treating gastritis. Adopting healthy eating habits may dramatically reduce symptoms and facilitate recovery. When dealing with gastritis, it is essential to eat meals that are mild on the stomach lining and reduce inflammation.

First and foremost, try adding more fruits and vegetables to your diet. These are high in vitamins, minerals, and antioxidants, which may aid in decreasing inflammation and promote overall digestive health. Choose fruits with low acidity, such as bananas, apples, and pears, which are simple to digest.

Similarly, veggies like carrots, spinach, and sweet potatoes are easy on the stomach while providing critical nutrients.

Whole grains are another essential dietary component for treating gastritis. They are high in fiber, which assists digestion and encourages regular bowel motions. Choose whole grains such as brown rice, quinoa, and whole wheat bread over processed grains, which may worsen inflammation.

Lean proteins help to heal and maintain the stomach lining. Include sources including skinless chicken, fish, tofu, and lentils in your meals. These protein sources are simpler to digest than fatty meats, which may help avoid further inflammation.

Additionally, it is critical to keep hydrated by drinking enough water throughout the day. Avoiding substances that might worsen gastritis, such as alcohol and caffeinated drinks, is also recommended. Instead, to ease the stomach, drink herbal teas, coconut water, or diluted fruit juice.

Finally, be cautious of food quantities and meal times. Eating smaller, more frequent meals can help to prevent stomach overload and discomfort. Eat at regular intervals and avoid large meals before bedtime, as lying down soon after eating can worsen symptoms.

Stress Management Techniques

Stress can worsen gastritis symptoms by raising stomach acid levels and causing inflammation. Incorporating stress management techniques into your daily routine can help to reduce these effects and promote healing.

Deep breathing exercises are an efficient stress-management method. Deep breathing is accomplished by slowly inhaling through your nose, allowing your abdomen to fully expand, and then slowly exhaling through your mouth. This can help to trigger the body's relaxation response and lower stress levels.

Regular physical activity is another great way to reduce stress and improve overall health. Spend at least 30 minutes per day doing activities you enjoy, such as walking, yoga, or swimming. Exercise produces endorphins, which are natural mood enhancers that can help reduce stress and anxiety.

Mindfulness and meditation techniques can also be useful for stress reduction. Take a few minutes each day to sit quietly and concentrate on your breath, or to practice guided meditation techniques. This can help to relax the mind, increase emotional resilience, and alleviate stress-related symptoms.

It is critical to prioritize self-care and allocate time for activities that bring you joy and relaxation. Finding ways to unwind and recharge, whether through reading, nature walks, or hobbies, is critical for stress management and overall health.

Avoiding Irritants

Certain foods and beverages can worsen gastritis symptoms by irritating the stomach lining. Avoiding these irritants can help to alleviate discomfort and promote healing.

Spicy foods are one of the most common irritants, as they increase stomach acid and aggravate inflammation. To prevent gastritis symptoms from worsening, limit or avoid spicy foods like curries, hot sauces, and chili peppers.

Similarly, acidic foods and beverages can irritate the stomach lining, worsening gastritis. Citrus fruits, tomatoes, and citrus juices are acidic foods that should be consumed in moderation or avoided entirely. Choose milder alternatives such as bananas, melons, and green vegetables.

Fatty and fried foods have also been shown to worsen gastritis symptoms by slowing digestion and increasing the risk of acid reflux. Limit your intake of greasy foods like fried chicken, burgers, and French fries, and instead use lighter cooking methods like baking, grilling, or steaming.

Alcohol and caffeinated beverages are known to irritate the stomach lining and increase acid production. Limit your intake of alcohol and caffeinated beverages such as coffee, tea, and soda, and instead drink herbal teas or water.

Finally, avoid eating large meals close to bedtime, as lying down can increase the risk of acid reflux and worsen gastritis symptoms. Allow at least two to three hours between your last meal and bedtime to ensure proper digestion and reduce discomfort.

Importance Of Adequate Sleep

Getting enough sleep is essential for treating gastritis and improving overall health and well-being. During sleep, the body goes through necessary processes that help digestion, repair tissues, and regulate hormone levels.

Chronic sleep deprivation can disrupt these processes and worsen gastritis symptoms by elevating stress hormones and inflammation. Aim for seven to nine hours of quality sleep per night to promote digestive health and lower the risk of gastritis flare-ups.

Creating a consistent sleep schedule can help regulate your body's internal clock and improve sleep quality. To promote a consistent sleep-wake cycle, go to bed and wake up at the same times every day, including weekends.

Create a soothing bedtime routine to signal to your body that it's time to unwind and prepare for sleep. This could include reading, taking a warm bath, or practicing relaxation techniques like deep breathing or meditation.

Maintain a dark, quiet, and comfortably cool bedroom to promote restful sleep. Invest in a comfortable mattress and pillows to improve your sleeping posture and reduce discomfort.

Avoid stimulating activities and electronic devices, such as smartphones and computers, in the hour before bedtime, as they can disrupt your ability to fall asleep. Instead, engage in relaxing activities that will prepare your mind and body for sleep.

Prioritizing adequate sleep and developing healthy sleep habits can help your body's natural healing processes while also reducing the frequency and severity of gastritis symptoms.

CHAPTER 5

Medications For Gastritis

Antacids

Antacids are over-the-counter medications used to treat gastric symptoms such as heartburn and indigestion. These medications work by neutralizing stomach acid, which relieves irritation and inflammation in the stomach lining.

Aluminum hydroxide, magnesium hydroxide, or calcium carbonate are key components of antacids. These substances react with the excess acid in the stomach to produce salts and water. This reaction helps to raise the pH level in the stomach, which reduces acidity and relieves symptoms.

Antacids come in several forms, including tablets, chewable tablets, and liquid suspensions. They are generally safe for short-term use and offer quick relief from symptoms. However, prolonged use of antacids may result in side effects such as constipation or diarrhea, so it is critical to use them as prescribed by a healthcare professional.

Proton Pump Inhibitors (Ppis)

Medication known as proton pump inhibitors (PPIs) lowers the production of stomach acid. They are extremely effective in treating gastritis caused by high acid levels or conditions like gastroesophageal reflux disease (GERD).

PPIs work by inhibiting the proton pumps in the stomach lining, which produce acid. PPIs effectively reduce acid in the stomach by blocking these pumps, thereby alleviating symptoms and promoting stomach lining healing.

Omeprazole, esomeprazole, lansoprazole, and pantoprazole are among the most commonly prescribed PPIs. These medications are typically taken orally, as tablets or capsules, once per day before a meal.

While PPIs are generally safe and well tolerated, prolonged use may increase the risk of bone fractures or vitamin B12 deficiency. It is critical to use PPIs under the supervision of a healthcare professional and adhere to their recommendations for dosage and duration of treatment.

H2 Receptor Blockers

H2 receptor blockers, also called H2 antagonists, are another type of medication used to reduce stomach acid production. They function by inhibiting the action of histamine, a chemical in the body that stimulates the production of stomach acid.

H2 receptor blockers reduce acid production by inhibiting histamine's effects on the stomach lining, reducing irritation and inflammation.

Ranitidine, famotidine, and cimetidine are among the most commonly prescribed H2 receptor blockers. These medications are available over the counter or by prescription and are typically taken orally in tablet or liquid form.

H2 receptor blockers are generally well tolerated, but as with PPIs, long-term use may increase the risk of pneumonia or vitamin B12 deficiency. These medications must be taken exactly as prescribed by a healthcare professional, and any concerns or potential side effects should be discussed with them.

Antibiotics (For H. Pylori Infection)

Antibiotics are frequently prescribed to treat gastritis caused by Helicobacter pylori (H. pylori) bacteria.

H. pylori infection is a common cause of gastritis and, if left untreated, can progress to more serious complications such as peptic ulcers or stomach cancer. Antibiotics work by targeting and killing bacteria, thus removing the underlying cause of inflammation.

Frequently prescribed antibiotics for H. Clarithromycin, amoxicillin, metronidazole, and tetracycline are among the medications used to treat H. pylori infections. These antibiotics are typically used in conjunction with other medications, such as PPIs or H2 receptor blockers, to ensure effective treatment.

It is critical to finish the entire course of antibiotics as prescribed by a healthcare professional, even if symptoms improve before the course is completed. Failure to do so may cause the bacteria to become resistant to antibiotics, making future treatment difficult.

In addition to antibiotics, other medications may be prescribed to help manage gastritis symptoms, such as pain relievers or stomach lining protectants. You must collaborate closely with a healthcare provider in order to create a thorough treatment plan that is customized to meet your individual requirements.

CHAPTER 6

Herbal Remedies And Natural Treatments

Aloe Vera

Aloe vera, a succulent plant, has been used medicinally for centuries. Its gel-like substance, which is found in the fleshy part of its leaves, contains vitamins, minerals, amino acids, and enzymes that are thought to have medicinal properties. Aloe vera is commonly recommended for gastritis due to its anti-inflammatory and soothing effects on the stomach lining.

You can take aloe vera for gastritis relief in the form of juice or gel. Aloe vera juice is commercially available in health food stores, and the gel can be extracted from fresh aloe vera leaves. It's important to note that while aloe vera can help some people with gastritis, others may experience side effects like diarrhea or abdominal cramps. It is best to begin with a small dose and monitor your body's response.

Ginger

Ginger is a popular spice and medicinal herb, known for its anti-inflammatory and nausea-reducing properties. It contains bioactive compounds such as gingerol, which has been shown to help alleviate gastritis symptoms by reducing inflammation in the stomach lining and improving digestion.

There are several ways to incorporate ginger into your diet to alleviate gastritis symptoms. You can make ginger tea by steeping fresh ginger slices in hot water, or you can mix grated ginger into your meals and smoothies. Some people get relief from chewing on a small piece of raw ginger or taking ginger supplements in capsule form. However, before using ginger supplements, you should consult with a healthcare professional, especially if you are taking medication or have any underlying health conditions.

Licorice Root

Licorice root, derived from the root of the Glycyrrhiza glabra plant, has been used in traditional medicine for a variety of health benefits, including the ability to treat digestive issues such as gastritis. It contains glycyrrhizin and flavonoids, which have anti-inflammatory and protective properties for the stomach lining.

Licorice root can be consumed in a variety of forms, including tea, supplements, and chewable tablets. Licorice tea is made by steeping dried licorice root in hot water for a few minutes. However, licorice root should be consumed with caution because excessive or prolonged use can cause side effects such as high blood pressure, potassium depletion, and hormone imbalances. Licorice root should also be avoided by people who have hypertension, kidney disease, or are pregnant.

Probiotics

Probiotics are live microorganisms that can provide health benefits when consumed in sufficient quantities. They are commonly known as "good" or "friendly" bacteria due to their beneficial effects on the digestive system. Probiotics can help restore the balance of beneficial bacteria in the gut, which may be disrupted in conditions like gastritis.

Probiotics can be found naturally in fermented foods such as yogurt, kefir, sauerkraut, and kimchi, or they can be taken as supplements. When selecting a probiotic supplement, look for strains that have been specifically studied for their efficacy in treating digestive issues like gastritis, such as Lactobacillus and Bifidobacterium species. To reap the full benefits, you must adhere to the manufacturer's recommended dosage instructions and maintain a consistent probiotic regimen. Furthermore, probiotics may not be appropriate for everyone, so consult with a healthcare professional before starting a new supplement regimen, especially if you are on medication or have underlying medical issues.

Each of these herbal remedies and natural treatments may provide relief from gastritis symptoms. However, you should use them with caution and consult with a healthcare professional before incorporating them into your treatment plan, especially if you have any underlying health conditions or are taking medications. By combining these natural remedies with lifestyle changes and conventional medical treatments as needed, you can effectively manage gastritis and improve your overall digestive health.

CHAPTER 7

Preventing Gastritis Flare-Ups

Maintaining A Healthy Diet

Maintaining a healthy diet is essential for avoiding gastritis flare-ups and improving overall digestive health. When it comes to diet, it's critical to prioritize foods that are gentle on the stomach lining and lower inflammation. Eat a diet high in whole grains, fruits, vegetables, and lean meats. These foods contain essential nutrients and fiber while being easily digestible.

Fiber-rich foods, such as fruits, vegetables, and whole grains, aid digestion and prevent constipation, which can aggravate gastritis symptoms. Incorporating probiotic-rich foods such as yogurt, kefir, and sauerkraut can also promote the growth of beneficial bacteria in the gut, thereby improving digestive health.

On the other hand, it is critical to avoid foods that can cause inflammation and irritate the stomach lining. Spicy, fried, acidic foods (such as citrus fruits and tomatoes), and fatty foods should be limited or avoided entirely. These foods can exacerbate gastritis symptoms, causing discomfort and inflammation.

In addition to selecting the right foods, consider portion sizes and meal timing. Eating smaller, more frequent meals throughout the day can help prevent stomach overload and reduce the likelihood of flare-ups. It's also best to avoid eating large meals right before bedtime, as lying down after eating can increase the risk of acid reflux and worsen gastritis symptoms.

Individuals can significantly reduce their risk of gastritis flare-ups and improve their digestive health by eating a balanced and nutritious diet that focuses on whole foods and avoids triggers.

Stress Reduction Strategies

Stress is a common trigger for gastritis flare-ups because it disrupts digestive processes and causes inflammation in the stomach lining. As a result, implementing effective stress reduction strategies is critical for managing gastritis and avoiding recurrence.

Deep breathing, meditation, and yoga are among the most effective stress-reduction techniques. These practices encourage relaxation, reduce muscle tension, and calm the mind, making them useful tools for stress management and overall well-being.

Regular exercise is another effective stress-management technique that can help people with gastritis. Physical activity produces endorphins, which are natural mood enhancers that help reduce stress and anxiety. Exercise also improves circulation and digestion, which can lead to better overall digestive health.

Incorporating hobbies and activities that bring joy and fulfillment can also aid in stress reduction. Whether it's spending time outside, engaging in a creative outlet like painting or gardening, or simply spending quality time with loved ones, finding activities that provide relaxation and enjoyment can have a significant impact on stress levels and overall health.

Furthermore, prioritizing self-care practices such as adequate sleep, relaxation baths, and massage therapy can aid in stress management and reduce the likelihood of gastritis flare-ups.

Individuals who incorporate stress reduction strategies into their daily routine can better manage their stress levels, support their digestive health, and lower their risk of gastritis flare-ups.

Limiting Alcohol And Caffeine Intake

Alcohol and caffeine are known stomach lining irritants that can exacerbate gastritis symptoms, so they should be limited or avoided to prevent flare-ups.

Alcohol irritates the stomach lining and raises stomach acid levels, which can cause inflammation and irritation. Even moderate alcohol consumption can cause symptoms of gastritis, including abdominal pain, nausea, and indigestion. To prevent flare-ups and promote digestive health, it is best to limit or avoid alcohol consumption entirely.

Similarly, caffeine can increase stomach acid production while relaxing the muscles that control food passage from the stomach to the intestines, causing increased irritation and inflammation in people with gastritis. Caffeine is commonly found in coffee, tea, soda, and energy drinks. While some people can tolerate small amounts of caffeine without experiencing symptoms, others may find that even one cup of coffee worsens their gastritis. To avoid flare-ups, it's important to monitor and limit caffeine consumption.

Individuals with gastritis can replace alcohol and caffeine with hydrating, non-irritating beverages like herbal teas, infused water, and non-acidic fruit juices. These beverages provide hydration without irritating the stomach lining, making them good choices for people trying to avoid gastritis flare-ups.

Individuals can reduce their risk of gastritis flare-ups and improve their digestive health by limiting their consumption of alcohol and caffeine and opting for hydrating alternatives.

Avoiding Smoking

Smoking is a major risk factor for gastritis and can exacerbate symptoms in those who already have the condition. Cigarette smoke contains many harmful chemicals that can irritate the stomach lining and cause inflammation, resulting in discomfort and potentially serious complications.

Nicotine, a key component of tobacco smoke, can weaken the lower esophageal sphincter (LES), the muscle that controls food flow from the esophagus to the stomach. When the LES is weakened, stomach acid can reflux into the esophagus, causing heartburn and exacerbating gastritis symptoms.

Furthermore, smoking interferes with the healing process of the stomach lining, making it more difficult for people with gastritis to recover from inflammation and damage.

Smoking regularly increases the risk of developing complications such as peptic ulcers and stomach cancer.

Quitting smoking is critical for people with gastritis because it reduces inflammation, promotes healing, and prevents flare-ups. While quitting smoking can be difficult, there are numerous resources and support systems available to help people quit, such as nicotine replacement therapy, counseling, and support groups.

Quitting smoking and avoiding secondhand smoke can significantly reduce the risk of gastritis flare-ups while also improving overall digestive health.

CHAPTER 8

Complications Of Gastritis

Peptic Ulcers

Peptic ulcers are a common complication of gastritis that causes sores or lesions in the stomach or upper part of the small intestine. These ulcers can be caused by erosion of the protective lining as a result of gastritis-induced inflammation. Common risk factors for the development of peptic ulcers include Helicobacter pylori (H. pylori) infection, prolonged use of nonsteroidal anti-inflammatory drugs (NSAIDs), excessive alcohol consumption, and smoking.

When the stomach's protective mucosal barrier fails, acidic digestive juices and the presence of H. pylori bacteria can cause damage to the underlying tissues, resulting in ulcers.

Symptoms of a peptic ulcer include abdominal pain, bloating, nausea, vomiting, and black or bloody stools. If left untreated, peptic ulcers can cause serious complications such as bleeding, perforation (a hole in the stomach wall), and obstruction (blockage) in the digestive system.

Peptic ulcers are typically treated with a combination of medications designed to reduce stomach acid production and eradicate H. pylori infection (if present) while also protecting the stomach and intestine lining. Proton pump inhibitors (PPIs), H2-receptor antagonists, antibiotics, and antacids are commonly used to treat peptic ulcers. In severe cases, endoscopic therapy or surgery may be necessary to stop bleeding or repair perforations.

Gastric Cancer

Gastric cancer, also known as stomach cancer, is a serious complication of chronic gastritis, particularly if it is not treated or managed properly. Chronic inflammation of the gastric mucosa can cause genetic mutations and changes in cellular structure, raising the risk of malignant transformation and gastric cancer.

Gastric cancer is caused by a variety of factors, including H. infection. pylori bacteria, chronic gastritis, smoking, a diet rich in smoked, pickled, or salty foods, and certain genetic predispositions. Early-stage gastric cancer may not produce noticeable symptoms, but as the disease progresses, patients may experience persistent abdominal pain, unexplained weight loss, difficulty swallowing, vomiting, and blood in the stool.

Gastric cancer is typically diagnosed using a combination of imaging tests, including endoscopy, biopsy, and imaging scans (CT scan, MRI, or PET scan), to determine the extent and spread of the cancer. Gastric cancer treatment options may include surgery to remove the tumor, chemotherapy, radiation therapy, targeted therapy, and immunotherapy, depending on the cancer's stage and location.

Anemia

Anemia is a condition characterized by a lack of red blood cells or hemoglobin in the blood, which can develop as a result of chronic gastritis. Chronic inflammation of the stomach lining can impair the absorption of essential nutrients such as iron, vitamin B12, and folic acid, resulting in decreased red blood cell production and anemia.

Anemia symptoms vary depending on the severity and underlying cause but may include fatigue, weakness, shortness of breath, pale skin, dizziness, and headaches. Anemia is typically diagnosed through a blood test that measures hemoglobin and red blood cell levels while also identifying any underlying deficiencies or conditions that contribute to the anemia.

Treatment for anemia caused by gastritis frequently focuses on addressing the root cause of the deficiency. This could include changing your diet to include iron-rich foods like red meat, poultry, fish, leafy green vegetables, and fortified cereals, as well as taking iron, vitamin B12, or folic acid supplements as needed. In some cases, if malabsorption is severe, intravenous iron or vitamin B12 injections may be prescribed.

Malabsorption

Malabsorption is the impaired absorption of nutrients from the gastrointestinal tract, which can occur as a side effect of gastritis caused by inflammation and damage to the stomach and intestine linings. Chronic gastritis, particularly autoimmune or atrophic gastritis, can destroy the gastric mucosa and cause the loss of essential digestive enzymes, reducing nutrient absorption such as vitamins, minerals, fats, and carbohydrates.

Diarrhea, weight loss, abdominal bloating and discomfort, flatulence, and deficiencies in essential nutrients such as vitamin B12, iron, calcium, and fat-soluble vitamins (A, D, E, and K) are examples of common malabsorption symptoms. Malabsorption is commonly diagnosed using a combination of blood tests, stool tests, imaging studies, and, in some cases, endoscopic procedures to assess the extent of gastrointestinal damage.

Treatment for malabsorption caused by gastritis aims to correct nutrient deficiencies and improve gastrointestinal function. This may include dietary changes, such as eliminating trigger foods that aggravate symptoms and incorporating easily digestible, nutrient-dense foods. Supplementation with vitamins, minerals, and digestive enzymes may also be required to address deficiencies and improve nutrient absorption. In severe cases, medications to reduce inflammation and promote gastrointestinal healing may be prescribed, along with close monitoring by healthcare providers to optimize treatment outcomes.

Individuals can take proactive steps to manage their condition and reduce the risk of serious complications by understanding these potential gastritis complications, as well as their associated symptoms, risk factors, diagnosis, and treatment options.

Early detection and intervention are critical for preventing the progression of gastritis-related complications and improving overall gastrointestinal health and well-being.

CHAPTER 9

Gastritis In Special Populations

Gastritis In Children

Gastritis in children can be concerning for parents because it causes inflammation of the stomach lining, which can cause discomfort and other symptoms. Understanding the causes, symptoms, and management of gastritis in children is critical to ensuring their health.

Causes

Several factors can lead to gastritis in children. These include bacterial infections, particularly Helicobacter pylori, which is a common cause of gastritis in children and adults. Other potential causes include autoimmune disorders, long-term use of nonsteroidal anti-inflammatory drugs (NSAIDs), specific medications, and dietary factors.

Symptoms

Recognizing the symptoms of gastritis in children is critical for early intervention. Symptoms can range from abdominal pain or discomfort to nausea, vomiting, bloating, loss of appetite, and, in some cases, blood in vomit or stool. Children may exhibit irritability or mood changes as a result of their discomfort.

Diagnosis

Children's gastritis is frequently diagnosed using a combination of medical history, physical examination, and diagnostic tests. These tests may include blood tests to detect H. pylori infection, stool tests to detect blood in the stool, and imaging studies such as upper gastrointestinal endoscopy to visualize the stomach lining and collect biopsies for further testing.

Treatment

Treatment for gastritis in children aims to alleviate symptoms, address underlying causes, and prevent complications. This could include medications like proton pump inhibitors (PPIs) to reduce stomach acid production and antibiotics to eliminate H. If H. pylori infection is present, avoid triggers such as certain foods or medications that may aggravate symptoms. In severe cases, hospitalization with intravenous fluids may be required.

Prevention

Children's gastritis can be prevented by promoting a healthy lifestyle and reducing risk factors. Encourage proper hygiene, including handwashing, to help prevent bacterial infections. Furthermore, limiting NSAID use and eating a well-balanced diet can help children's stomach health.

Gastritis During Pregnancy

Gastritis during pregnancy presents unique challenges due to hormonal changes and physiological adaptations in the body. Effective management of gastritis during pregnancy is critical for both maternal and fetal health.

Causes

The causes of gastritis during pregnancy may differ from those in non-pregnant people. Hormonal changes, particularly increased progesterone levels, can cause stomach muscles to relax and gastric motility to decrease, potentially contributing to gastritis. Dietary changes, stress levels, and pre-existing gastrointestinal conditions can all exacerbate pregnancy symptoms.

Symptoms

Pregnant women with gastritis may experience heartburn, nausea, vomiting, bloating, and abdominal discomfort. These symptoms vary in severity and can be exacerbated by certain foods or stressors. Pregnant women must communicate any discomfort or unusual symptoms to their healthcare provider for proper management.

Diagnosis

Gastritis during pregnancy must be diagnosed with care, taking into account both symptoms and risk factors. To diagnose H, healthcare providers may conduct a physical examination, review medical history, and recommend diagnostic tests such as upper gastrointestinal endoscopy or blood tests. pylori infection or another underlying cause.

Treatment

Gastritis during pregnancy necessitates a cautious approach to protect both the mother and the developing fetus. Dietary changes, stress-reduction techniques, and elevating the head while sleeping can all help to relieve symptoms. Healthcare providers may also prescribe medications such as antacids or H2-receptor antagonists while keeping pregnancy safety in mind.

Gastritis In The Elderly

Gastritis in the elderly poses special challenges due to age-related changes in the gastrointestinal tract, comorbidities, and polypharmacy. Effective gastritis management in the elderly necessitates a comprehensive approach that takes into account their unique needs and health status.

Causes

Gastritis in the elderly can be caused by a variety of factors, including chronic Helicobacter pylori infection, long-term use of NSAIDs or corticosteroids, excessive alcohol consumption, and underlying medical conditions like autoimmune disorders or gastrinoma. Age-related changes in the gastric mucosa, as well as decreased gastric acid secretion, can predispose the elderly to gastritis.

Symptoms

Elderly people with gastritis may experience abdominal pain, indigestion, bloating, nausea, vomiting, and loss of appetite. However, symptoms can be subtle or nonspecific, making diagnosis difficult. Healthcare providers should have a high level of suspicion for gastritis in elderly patients, particularly those with multiple comorbidities.

Diagnosis

In the elderly, diagnosing gastritis may necessitate a combination of clinical examination, medical history review, and diagnostic tests. Upper gastrointestinal endoscopy with biopsy may be performed by a healthcare provider to visualize the stomach lining and detect inflammation or lesions.

Blood tests can detect H. pylori infection or other underlying conditions may also be present.

Treatment

The goal of treating gastritis in the elderly is to relieve symptoms, promote gastric mucosal healing, and avoid complications. This could include medications like proton pump inhibitors (PPIs) to reduce gastric acid secretion and antibiotics to eliminate H. If H. pylori infection is present, lifestyle changes such as dietary changes and stress reduction techniques should be implemented. When prescribing medications to elderly patients, healthcare providers should be aware of potential drug interactions and side effects.

Prevention

Preventing gastritis in the elderly entails addressing modifiable risk factors and encouraging healthy aging.

Regular medical check-ups, avoiding excessive alcohol consumption, and limiting the use of NSAIDs and other medications that can irritate the stomach lining can all help prevent gastritis. Additionally, maintaining a balanced diet rich in fruits, vegetables, and fiber can help elderly people with their gastrointestinal health.

CHAPTER 10

Living Well With Gastritis

Long-Term Management Strategies

Effective gastritis management necessitates a multifaceted approach that addresses both acute symptoms and long-term management. Long-term strategies include making lifestyle changes to reduce inflammation and discomfort in the stomach lining. Adopting a healthy diet is an important step. This includes avoiding spicy, acidic, and fatty foods, which can worsen gastritis symptoms. Instead, aim to incorporate more fruits, vegetables, whole grains, and lean proteins into your diet.

Stress management is also an important aspect of long-term management. Stress can exacerbate gastritis symptoms, so it is critical to find ways to relax and unwind.

This could include practicing mindfulness or meditation, getting regular exercise, or pursuing hobbies that bring joy and relaxation.

In addition to lifestyle changes, some people may benefit from long-term treatment for gastritis symptoms. This could include antacids to neutralize stomach acid, proton pump inhibitors (PPIs) to reduce acid production or stomach lining protection medications.

Regular check-ins with a healthcare provider are essential for long-term management. They can monitor your condition, adjust medications as needed, and offer advice on how to effectively manage symptoms.

Coping With Flare-Ups

Despite your best efforts, flare-ups of gastritis symptoms may occur on occasion. When this happens, you must have effective coping strategies in place. First, listen to your body and identify any triggers that may have contributed to the flare-up. This could include dietary mistakes, stress, or certain medications.

During a flare-up, your stomach needs time to rest and heal. This could include sticking to bland, easily digestible foods, avoiding alcohol and caffeine, and staying hydrated. Antacids and other over-the-counter medications can provide temporary relief from symptoms such as heartburn and indigestion.

In addition to managing physical symptoms, it is critical to prioritize self-care during flare-ups. This could include practicing relaxation techniques, getting enough sleep, and seeking support from friends and family.

If flare-ups become frequent or severe, do not hesitate to contact your healthcare provider for advice. They can help you identify underlying causes and adjust your treatment plan accordingly.

Support Networks And Resources

Living with gastritis can be difficult, but you do not have to face it alone. Creating a support network of friends, family, and healthcare professionals can be extremely helpful and encouraging. Don't be afraid to turn to your loved ones for emotional support, whether it's a listening ear or practical help with daily tasks.

In addition to personal support networks, there are resources available to help you manage gastritis successfully. This could include educational materials from credible sources, online support groups, or community-based programs. These resources can provide useful information, practical advice, and a sense of community among those facing similar challenges.

Remember that seeking help demonstrates strength, not weakness. Don't be afraid to ask for help when you need it, whether from loved ones or professional resources.

Importance Of Regular Check-Ups

Regular check-ups with your doctor are essential for effectively managing gastritis over time. These check-ups allow your doctor to monitor your condition, track any changes in symptoms, and adjust your treatment plan as necessary.

During check-ups, your healthcare provider may order blood tests, stool tests, or imaging studies to evaluate the health of your stomach lining and identify any underlying causes of your gastritis.

Regular check-ups not only monitor your physical health but also allow you to discuss any concerns or questions you may have about your condition. Your healthcare provider can advise you on how to manage your symptoms, make lifestyle changes, and deal with any other gastritis-related issues.

By getting regular check-ups and being proactive about your health, you can better manage gastritis and reduce its impact on your life. If you have any concerns or notice any changes in your symptoms, please schedule an appointment with your healthcare provider right away.

CONCLUSION

In conclusion, gastritis is a complex condition that necessitates attention and care. Through this investigation, it becomes clear that gastritis is a group of disorders, each with its own set of triggers, symptoms, and treatment strategies. Acute inflammation caused by infections such as H. Gastritis manifests in a variety of ways, ranging from chronic irritation caused by lifestyle factors such as excessive alcohol consumption or long-term use of nonsteroidal anti-inflammatory drugs.

The value of early detection and intervention cannot be overstated. Early detection, often achieved through endoscopic examination and histological analysis, enables targeted treatment, preventing complications such as peptic ulcers, bleeding, and, in severe cases, gastric cancer.

Treatment approaches differ depending on the underlying cause, but they typically include a combination of medications, dietary changes, and lifestyle modifications. Acid-suppressing medications, such as proton pump inhibitors (PPIs), relieve symptoms by lowering stomach acid production, whereas antibiotics may be required to treat bacterial infections like H. pylori. Lifestyle changes, such as dietary adjustments to avoid irritants, stress management techniques, and quitting smoking and excessive alcohol consumption, are critical for effectively managing gastritis.

However, the journey with gastritis does not end with medication. Long-term monitoring and follow-up are critical for determining treatment effectiveness, detecting recurrences, and addressing any remaining complications. Patient education and empowerment are also important aspects of gastritis management, allowing people to make informed decisions about their health and adopt habits that promote gastric health.

In essence, while gastritis can be difficult to manage, it can be effectively treated with proper medical care, lifestyle changes, and ongoing support. Individuals can navigate gastritis with confidence and improve their overall well-being by taking a comprehensive approach that addresses the underlying causes and promotes gastric health.

THE END

www.ingramcontent.com/pod-product-compliance
Lightning Source LLC
Chambersburg PA
CBHW070315230526
45470CB00002B/890